Beginner Weight Loss Tips

Eat to Live

By Cathy Wilson
Copyright © 2014

Income Disclaimer

This book contains business strategies, marketing methods and other business advice that, regardless of my own results and experience, may not produce the same results (or any results) for you. I make absolutely no guarantee, expressed or implied, that by following the advice below you will make any money or improve current profits, as there are several factors and variables that come into play regarding any given business.

Primarily, results will depend on the nature of the product or business model, the conditions of the marketplace, the experience of the individual, and situations and elements that are beyond your control.

As with any business endeavor, you assume all risk related to investment and money based on your own discretion and at your own potential expense.

Liability Disclaimer

By reading this book, you assume all risks associated with using the advice given below, with a full understanding that you, solely, are responsible for anything that may occur as a result of putting this information into action in any way, and regardless of your interpretation of the advice.

You further agree that our company cannot be held responsible in any way for the success or failure of your business as a result of the information presented in this book. It is your responsibility to conduct your own due diligence regarding the safe and successful operation of your business if you intend to apply any of our information in any way to your business operations.

Terms of Use

You are given a non-transferable, "personal use" license to this book. You cannot distribute it or share it with other individuals.

Also, there are no resale rights or private label rights granted when purchasing this book. In other words, it's for your own personal use only.

Beginner Weight Loss Tips

Eat to Live

By Cathy Wilson

Table of Contents

Introduction 9

Protein 13

Carbohydrates 17

Good Fats 23

Bad Fats 27

Essential Vitamins and Minerals 31

50 Nutrition Pointers for Success in Health 37

Final Thinking 53

Introduction

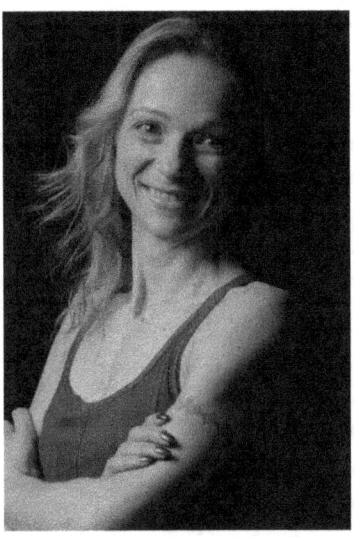

Hi. My name is Cathy Wilson and I am a fitness and nutrition expert. My focus in this beginner health and wellness book is to help you learn to love your body, drop weight safely and permanently, and gain the knowledge required to make you healthier FOR LIFE! Opening your mind to make positive life changes you can sustain and learn to love.

Fact is, most people give up on getting healthier because they either have expectations that are impossible, or they don't have the correct information and support to make the changes stick.

I will help you understand what good health is and how to attain it. Setting you up for success, so you have the base knowledge required to understand why you should eat certain things, how much your body needs to function, and when you should eat it. I will also talk about what happens if you don't make healthy food choices, while encouraging you to open your mind and truly understand how important your health really is.

I can lead you to the sources for change, give you all the information and encouragement you need to make healthy changes, but I can't make you implement them. That part is up to you. So if you are ready to open your mind to change for the better, I'm all set to deliver a fastball right down the center.

Pointers for Success in Health

What you eat influences your mood, weight, self-confidence, energy, physical composition and strength, and that's just the beginning. Your body knows what it requires to fight off dangerous free radicals; recognizes what nutrients it needs to keep you disease-free, energized to cover your physical requests, and to build your body and mind stronger.

Your thinking is very powerful, and by training your perspective to be positive, your life is going to be that much better.

The basics of what your body craves nutrient-wise to be healthy and functional are:

* Lean protein
* Complex carbohydrates
* Good fats
* Essential vitamins and minerals

That's about as general as I can get here, a starting point anyway. These nutrients are what your body craves to be healthy and happy. But that's only part of the equation. There's also regular physical activity, which I cover in another book!

FACT: In order for your internal systems to function effectively as a whole, you need exercise. Think of this as regular maintenance for your body. Sure you can run without it, but not very well. And since your body is going through the motions anyway, wouldn't you rather do this with less aches and pains, more energy, increased mobility, fewer serious diseases, and less trouble overall?

Starting Point

For success in nutrition you need to fuel your tank. In other words, you need to eat nutrient dense foods so your internal systems can run. The healthier you eat, the smoother your body will work. If you fill your body full of junk; bad fats, simple carbs and lots of sugar, you are going to look and feel like crap.

However, if you choose lean protein, lots of good carbs, good fats, and oodles of fruits and vegetables, your head will be sharper, body leaner, muscles stronger, tissues more resistant to disease, and you will be energized to the extreme.

Let's look at what you need to eat, how much, and when. Keeping in mind these amounts are general, because everybody is unique in their body composition, rate of metabolism, genetic makeup, lifestyle, amount they exercise, and overall health. Your health and wellness expert can help you fine tune your numbers if you like.

Protein

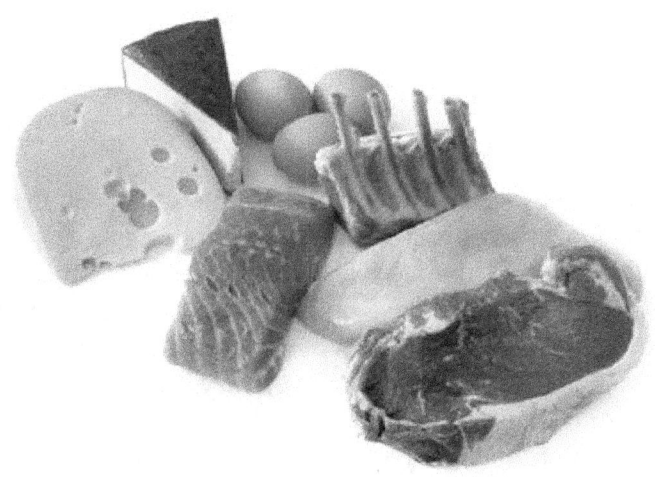

The What?

Protein is something you are going to find in every single cell in your body. Protein makes up most of your hair and nails, and your body uses protein to repair and create your tissues. Protein is critical in enzyme and hormone production, and is essential in bones, skin, blood, cartilage and muscles.

Your body needs large doses of protein and this makes it a macronutrient. Protein is something you need to give to your body on a regular basis because it can't make it, nor does it store protein. If you are trying to build muscle and not giving your body enough protein, it will simply break down and use your muscles to get it, which of course totally defeats the purpose of trying to build lean muscle in the first place!

The How Much?

So you can see that protein is vital to your health. Normally 2-3 servings of protein are required for the average woman each day. Of course if you are training hard, a little more may be required. For a serving size of meat just think of a deck of cards; 1 cup of milk, 3/4 cup of yogurt, or a 2x2 inch cube of cheese.

The When?

Lean protein is best eaten in small amounts with each meal. This will encourage your body to trust you that it will always be available for building muscle. Most people eat 3 meals a day. But if you can split these up into 5-6 mini-meals through-out the day, that's even better. What this does is ensure your body has a constant supply of fresh energy all day, which makes sense because you are constantly using your energy too. This will help curb your highs and lows, keeping your blood sugars constant. Experts also agree this will help decrease your risk of developing diabetes. With level blood sugar you'll also have less mood swings, and by eating small amounts regularly you'll also encourage your body to burn more calories in total.

Of course this isn't always possible, depending on your sched-ule. If you can swing it, that's only going to help better your health.

Health Alert - When it comes to portion sizes DO NOT use res-taurants as your base. Most restaurant portions are 3-4 times the size your body needs. So a trick when eating out is to ask for a take-out container even before they bring your meal. When your meal arrives take at least half of it and put it straight into the container without thinking about it. If you are like me, what's on my plate will get eaten whether I'm hungry or not. If I've already got the extra put away, I'm not going to wolf it down, and lunch is made for tomorrow!

Protein Sources

* White Meat Poultry - White meat has less fat than dark meat. Make sure you take off the skin because it's pretty much all fat with zero nutrients.

* Fish/Seafood - Most fish is low in fat, which makes it a great choice for lean protein. Salmon has a little more fat but is recommended because of its incredibly healthy omega-3 fatty acids.

* Eggs - Ah, my favorite! If you are looking to go cheaper, eggs are your best protein bet. Experts have verified that an egg a day is okay, that's one serving.

* Cheese/Yogurt/Milk - With these protein sources you also get that added benefit of calcium, keeping your bones and teeth strong. If these protein sources are fortified with vitamin D, even better! It's best to opt for skim or low-fat if you can.

* Beans - Did you know just one cup of beans has the same amount of protein as an ounce of steak? But the best thing about beans is they are naturally low in fat and loaded with fiber. This helps to leave you with a "full" feeling and keeps you regular.

* Soy - Experts say that eating soy protein regularly will help to lower cholesterol. This is a lower fat protein source, which makes it a "heart healthy" choice.

* Other Sources - There are lots of different kinds of protein bars and drinks out there that can be used in a pinch. Be careful though to check the packaging and make sure they aren't loaded with unnecessary sugars, as many energy drinks are.

* Low-Fat Beef - Many people believe beef is fattening. If you eat too much of it then yes, beef can be fattening. But that goes

for anything you eat. Truth is, lean beef only has about one more gram of fat than a skinless chicken breast does. With lean beef you are also going to get a good dose of iron, B12, and zinc to start.

Health Alert - How you cook your protein and what toppings you add can change your protein source from healthy to un-healthy in a snap. When cooking your meats you want to broil, poach, bake, steam, or barbecue them. Steer clear of adding lots of oil or butter for flavor when salt and pepper or herbs and spices can do the trick. If you are sautéing a chicken for a stir-fry, use a little Pam instead of butter or oil. When you are barbecuing use barbecue sauce sparingly and don't top your meat with any cream sauce. Two tablespoons of butter is al-most 200 calories extra of ALL FAT, and not the "good" fat you want.

* Peanut Butter - Who doesn't like peanut butter? Well I guess there are some that are allergic to it. But if you are clear of that, peanut butter is another good source of protein. You do need to be careful though because it's high in fat. So if you are having a peanut butter sandwich on whole grain bread, make sure you just use a tablespoon of peanut butter.

My Thinking . . .

It's important to understand that protein is your friend. Gone are the days where people think protein makes you fat. This just isn't true. Any kind of food in extreme over a long period of time can add padding to your frame. What you need to do is make better lean protein choices and ensure you get 2-3 serv-ings a day. Don't forget that a serving size isn't what you get in a restaurant either. Giving your body adequate amounts of protein is going to help you better your health. Isn't that reason enough?

Carbohydrates

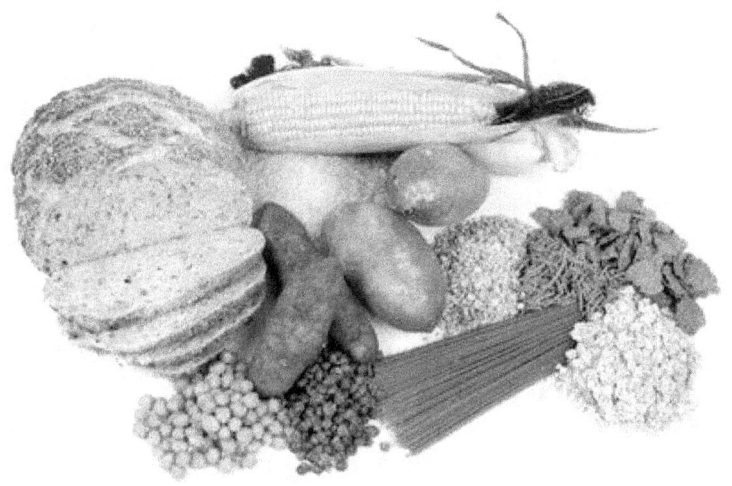

The What?

Carbohydrates are another macronutrient your body requires to function optimally. Actually, they are the most critical source of energy for your body. What happens is carbohydrates are broke down into blood sugar or glucose by your digestive juices. It's this sugar that your body uses to fuel the cells of your body. If you have excess sugar left over it gets stored away in your muscles and liver to be used later.

The two kinds of carbohydrates are simple and complex; just think "bad" and "good." There are a few exceptions to the rule here. Simple sugars are broken down easily and the energy provided is short-lived. Fruits and some vegetables, along with numerous milk and milk products are considered simple sugars. This also includes the sugars that are added during the refining process, including: cakes, pastries, cookies, sweets, and many other junky foods. The ones that taste great but do little for your health.

Complex carbohydrates are what you want to eat. These include whole grains, brown breads and rice, cereals, legumes, and starchy vegetables. They are loaded with fiber, take longer to digest and offer vital nutrients.

The point to remember here is that brown over white is how it's gotta be.

The How Much?

Experts agree you need about 50-65% of your daily calories from complex carbohydrates. But that would require us to do some math, and I'm just not up for that right now. An easier route that will keep things simple is to know that most adults need 6-11 servings every day. You'll probably do well aiming for 6-8 servings per day unless you are considerably larger than average, or are into some heavy exercising.

Don't worry. I'm not going to have you pulling out the scale to figure out exact serving sizes. We are going to go with the non-stressful eyeballing portions. Examples of portions are:

- 1 slice whole grain bread or 1/2 multigrain bagel
- 1/2 cup cooked cereal
- 1/2 cup cooked whole wheat pasta or rice
- 6-8 multigrain crackers
- Small banana
- 1 cup watermelon, cantaloupe, melon
- 1 apple or pear
- 10 grapes
- 1/2 cup fresh squeezed juice
- 1 cup yogurt
- 1/2 cup frozen vegetables

- Small potato

The When?

You should have 1-2 servings of complex carbohydrates with every meal. Try to spread your portions out evenly throughout the day. So maybe you'll have 1/2 cup oatmeal and fresh squeezed juice for breakfast. With lunch you might have whole grain bread with your sandwich and peas and a potato with dinner. Later you could have a banana as a snack.

Carbohydrate Sources

* All Vegetables - Veggies are very low in calories and high in essential vitamins, minerals and phytonutrients, which help better your health. Most are loaded with fiber, which leaves you feeling full longer. Sweet potatoes for instance, has protein, vitamin C, folate, calcium, and beta carotene.

Health Alert - It's important to eat healthy first to get control of sweet cravings. If you are hungry you should eat nutritious foods first, then have a sweet after if you still want. If you are starving and have a chocolate bar or bag of chips first, you are teaching your body to crave those unhealthy sweets whenever your tummy starts to rumble.

* Fruits - Most fruits are considered simple carbohydrates because they break down quickly in your system. So especially when trying to lose weight, veggies are a better option than fruit. Of course most people prefer fruit because it's so sweet. 2-3 pieces of fruit each day is plenty in most cases.

* Oatmeal - Packed with fiber, protein and numerous vitamins and mineral, and low in fat is what oatmeal's all about. Tasty too!

* Brown Rice and Whole Grain Pasta - Here you'll get whole-some goodness, lots of fiber, essential vitamins, and minerals. It's also low in fat.

* Whole Grain Bread, Pita, Bagels -

* Lentils, Yams, Sweet Potatoes -

Carbohydrates to Minimize

- White Pasta
- Instant Oatmeal
- White Rice
- Donuts
- Cakes
- Pastries
- Muffins
- Juices
- Sweets and Candies

Steer clear of processed carbohydrates if possible.

My Thinking . . .

There are all sorts of non-carb diets out there claiming to help people get fit and lose weight. I tend to stick with the diets that have a good track record and stay as close as possible to sim-ple. Let's rewind to back to the days of the cave man. They had no choice but to eat what nature provided. This is how they fueled their bodies with clean energy so they could thrive each day. Nature provided them with ample complex carbohydrates. So it just doesn't make sense that your body doesn't need this type of fuel now? Where we tend to step off course is when we opt for simple carbohydrates that don't usually provide the nu-trients we need. Things like while bread and pasta, pastries, and processed sweet treats. By giving your body adequate amounts of healthy whole grain products and other complex carbohydrates, you are going to give your body the energy it needs to work for you. Don't think about it, just do it!

Good Fats

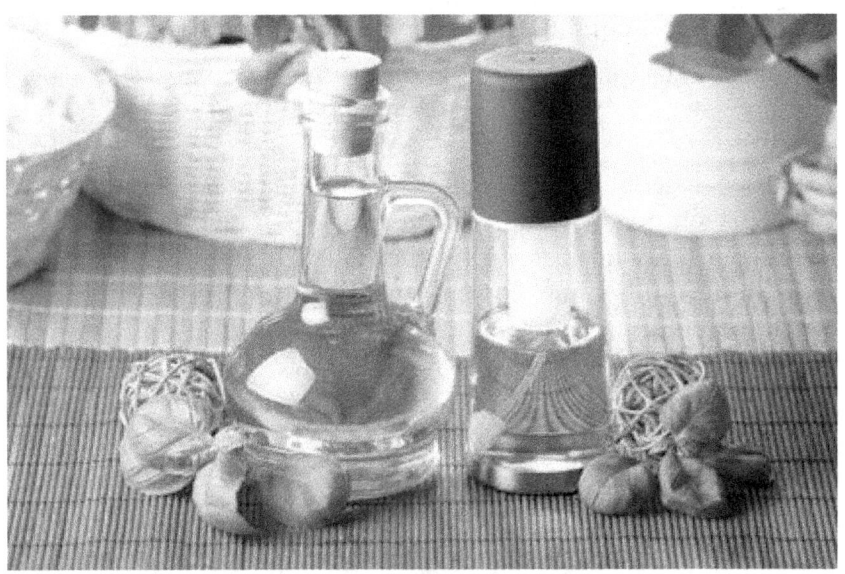

The What?

I understand it's pretty confusing to know which fats are okay for your body, and what ones to steer clear of. Most of us don't have an issue getting enough fat in our diet to be healthy. In fact, the majority of us get WAY too much. What's important is recognizing which types of fat you should be eating.

Health Alert - Getting rid of fat completely from your diet isn't going to solve our weight loss problems. The truth is you need fat and can't survive without it. Fats are part of a healthy diet; helping to keep your skin soft, providing essential fatty acids, energizing your body, and delivering important fat-soluble vitamins. Bottom line is you need fat to survive, where the problems and misconceptions arise are in what amount is required to be healthy and what types.

Experts recommend getting up to 35% of your daily calories from fat. That's not usually the issue though because we are a society that seems to get WAY too much fat. Chances are pretty good you get more fat than you need even when you are eating really, really, healthy. Focus on lowering your fat intake with healthier food choices, not worrying if you are getting enough.

Another misconception I want to clear up is that fat makes you fat. This simply isn't true. You get fat by eating more calories than your body utilizes, and it doesn't matter if it's protein, complex carbohydrates, or fat. If you get minimal exercise and eat too much food, you're going to gain weight. It's a combination of factors that leads you to pile on the pounds and get unhealthy.

The problem really isn't about carrying a little extra fat around. Medical issues arise because unhealthy lifestyle habits that lead to excessive fat, increase your risk for certain serious health diseases, including: diabetes, cancers, and cardiovascular disease. So getting healthy and lowering your body fat percentage is something you can do to get your head happy and body healthier.

Truth is, the wider your waistline, the greater chance you have of developing a life threatening condition.

Now we'll have a look at good fats and bad fats. Promise, I'll try to make this as simple as I can.

GOOD FATS

These are the unsaturated fats; monounsaturated and polyunsaturated fats. Eating them in moderation will help to lower cholesterol and decrease your risk of cardiovascular disease. These good fats are found mainly in vegetable oils, which are liquid at room temperature. Examples are coconut oil, olive oil, sunflower oil etc. Olives and avocados are great food sources.

Omega-3s are also important in good health, which you can get by eating two servings of fatty fish each week. Just think trout, catfish, salmon or mackerel. Keep in mind it's always better to try and get your omega-3s from food sources rather than supplements if possible. Your body will absorb them better. Monounsaturated fats also offer up the healthy antioxidant vitamin E, which helps protect the heart and is often missing in many diets. Good fats for this are peanuts, cashews, peanut oil, pumpkin seeds, almonds and avocados. Just be careful with the nuts because a handful is all you need in a serving. They are VERY high in calories and fat, and there is such thing as too much of a good thing.

The How Much?

Remember, all you really need is 10% of what you eat each day to be from fat calories. Seeing as 1 tbsp. of olive oil is approximately 100 calories of fat, it really doesn't take much to get your daily quota. Makes sense to open your mink to search for ways to decrease how much fat you are getting each day.

* Try a thin layer of peanut butter on your toast instead of butter.
* Try your dinner bread warm and naked instead of dipped in olive oil or slathered with butter.
* Use mustard or barbecue sauce on your sandwich instead of mayo or fatty dressings.
* Salad dressings are loaded with calories and fat. A trick is to get the dressing on the side and just drizzle on sparingly, or you can opt for fat-free options. Often the salads are loaded with fresh fruits and vegetables and don't even need dressing.
* When choosing pasta dishes, go for a tomato based dish rather than cream, and use cheese sparingly, a little goes a long way.

* When using a fry pan, just spray with cooking oil rather than using oil or butter. If you use oil, wipe the excess out of the pan with a paper towel.

Note - Don't expect to LOVE these adjustments right away. If you commit to doing it for at least six weeks, it will start to become a habit, your "new HEALTHY normal."

The When?

The ideal route is to eat fats sparingly and at every meal. This is especially important because some vitamins and minerals are absorbed better with good fats.

Good Fat Sources

Polyunsaturated

- Soybean and Sunflower Oil
- Fish and Corn Oil
- Various Seeds and Nuts
- Sunflower Oil

Monounsaturated

- Olives and Peanut Butter
- Olive and Canola Oil
- Avocado
- Walnut and Almond Oil
- Olives

Bad Fats

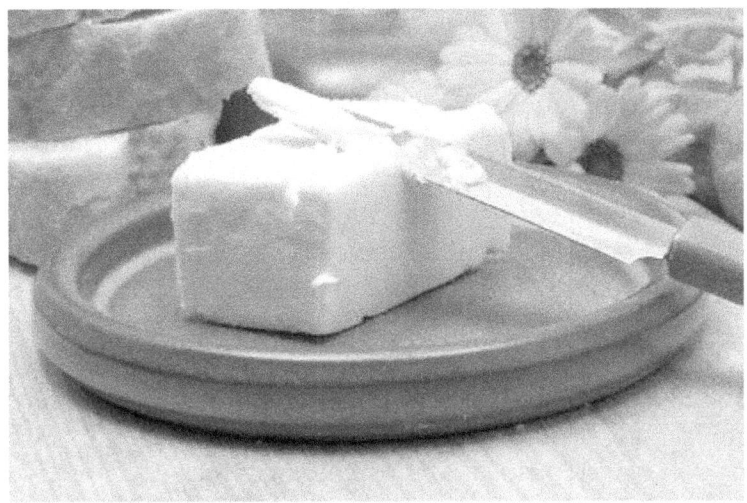

Saturated and Trans fatty acids shouldn't be eaten. They will contribute to high cholesterol levels, block arteries, and increase the chances of developing cardiovascular disease. Tran's fats are synthetic fats that are poisonous to your body – literally.

Saturated fats are found mainly in animal products. Things like meat, skin, eggs, and dairy. There are some oils, including coconut oil, that are considered saturated, but aren't "bad" for you, but that's a whole other book!

So why are these "bad" fats even legal, particularly the deadly Trans fats? Well because our world is driven by money and Trans fats is a fabricated version of fat that is cheaper than other fats. So when companies are looking to cut their production costs, particularly with sweets, pastries, muffins and other junk foods, they go for these unhealthy Trans fats. As well, Tran's fats have a longer shelf life and remain stable longer than other fats, something big food production companies want. How do you think a packaged muffin can last a month on the shelf? Eeek!

Now let's keep things realistic here. There's no need to get all freaked out if you do get some of these bad fats from time to time. Step by step you need to commit to making better food choices, and opting for foods with unsaturated fats instead of saturated. For instance, when cooking, use olive oil instead of butter in the pan. Better yet, use an oil spray instead, that's better for your waistline.

The big picture here, is that all fats need to be greatly reduced in order to get healthy. Understanding and managing fats will bring you one step closer to a happier healthier you.

The How Much?

Well you really don't want/need any bad fats. If you do get some, less than 5% of your total days' calories should come from bad fats.

The When?

Hmmm. Am I allowed to say never here?

Bad Fat Sources

- Lard or Butter
- Coconut Products (the jury is still out)
- Animal Skin
- Processed Lunch Meat

- Meat
- High-Fat Dairy Products
- Palm Oil
- Hydrogenated Oils (Partially)

My Thinking . . .

Fats are something you need to be healthy but there aren't many people that don't get enough in their regular eating. In fact, our societal problem is getting too much. So it's important to pay attention to what you are eating and learn to consciously make healthier food choices with less fat. When you do get fat it's important to opt for "good" fat. That's what your body needs and uses. One step at a time and you WILL get there.

Essential Vitamins and Minerals

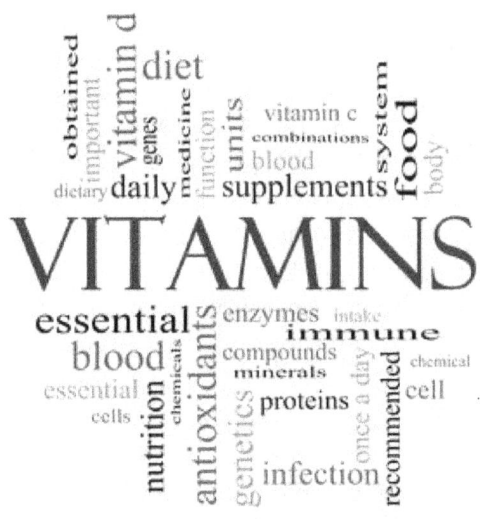

The What?

Vitamins and minerals are nutrients that help your body run effectively and efficiently. They are what keeps your body healthy.

Health Alert - Many people don't pay attention to the vitamins and minerals their body needs and just take a vitamin supplement instead. This is NOT a wise move because supplements aren't always readily absorbed by the body. Which means you could be taking a specific vitamin and it might just be shooting right through you. As well, there are nutrients that should be taken with a certain type of food in order to slow down the processing so your body can get the full benefit. An example is folic acid, which is best taken with your orange juice.

This doesn't mean you shouldn't ever take a supplement though. But the best route is to try and get all your vitamins and minerals from healthy food sources first.

VITAMINS

Now I don't want to overwhelm you here, but it's important that you understand a little bit about vitamins. This is only going to help you make better food choices so you do give your body what it craves for good health. Not perfect, just better.

There are 2 kinds of vitamins; water soluble and fat soluble. Water soluble vitamins are B complex, folic acid, and vitamin C. Fat soluble vitamins are dissolve in fat are include Vitamins D, E, K, and A.

The Benefits of Water Soluble Vitamins Are:

Vitamin C helps with antioxidant absorption, keeping skin and joints healthy, healing minor wounds, forming enzymes, and iron absorption. Citrus fruits and broccoli are excellent sources. And I'm sure you've heard of old-time sailors getting scurvy on sailing ships, where they have trouble healing, are tired and bleed from their skin? This is a sign of not getting enough Vitamin C.

Vitamin B Complex includes 10 nutrients. The main ones are Cyanocobalamin (B12), Niacin (B3), Thiamine (B1), Riboflavin (B2), Pyridoxine (B6), and Pantothenic Acid (B5). They help with your energy production, immune system, nervous system, and ability to absorb iron. If you don't give your body enough you can experience loss of hair, a swollen tongue, high heart rate, emotional issues, extreme tiredness, and lethargy. Great sources are whole grain breads and cereals, meat, and milk.

Folic acid is critical in DNA and RNA formation, which makes it very important in the diet of an expecting mother. A deficiency can mean serious birth defects for a baby, infertility, lack of energy, heart palpitations, paleness and extreme fatigue. Spinach, green beans, and Brussels sprouts are great sources.

MINERALS

There are macro, trace, and ultra trace minerals. To maintain your health, the body needs adequate doses of sodium, potassium, calcium, phosphorus, zinc, fluorine, and iron. The trace elements you need to be healthy are manganese, copper, molybdenum, iodine, and selenium.

Essential Minerals

Calcium ensures strong teeth and bones, and a healthy nervous system function. The best natural source is milk, and not getting enough can lead to stunted growth, a weak skeletal system, and dull hair and skin.

Iron is a mineral critical in red cell creation. You can get it by eating fish, eggs, and meat. If you have an iron deficiency you may feel extreme fatigue, have an increased heart rate, and weak nails.

Zinc is important in strengthening your immune system, for brain and body growth and development, speeding up the healing process for wounds, and bettering fertility. If you aren't getting enough you may be experiencing hair loss, diarrhea, skin swelling, slow growth, and a sore throat. This can be avoided by making sure you eat a balanced diet with milk, eggs, vegetables, grains, and lean meat.

Trace Minerals (most vital)

Iodine is something your body needs to develop and grow naturally because it helps make up your thyroid hormones. If you are deficient in iodine you may develop a goiter, which is a swollen or abnormally large thyroid gland. Iodine sources are fish from the ocean, milk, and iodized salt.

Chromium helps with glucose use. Losing weight and not being able to breakdown glucose are indicators you aren't getting enough. Eating a healthy diet including whole grains, nuts, and meat, will help ensure you get adequate amounts.

The How Much?

The best route for ensuring you get enough vitamins and minerals in your diet is to keep on eating healthy. Including plenty of lean meats, fruits and vegetables, low fat milk products, healthy whole grains, fish and eggs, ensures your body is getting what it needs to function optimally.

Note - If you are eating healthy and still experiencing some of the symptoms mentioned above, speak with your doctor to rule out serious issues.

The When?

Choosing a diverse range of nutritious foods regularly throughout the day, is key in getting healthy. The easiest way for you to get all the vitamins and minerals you need is to diversify, and eat healthy foods regularly.

Essential Vitamin and Mineral Sources

* Hard cheese, milk, yogurt
* Spinach, cereals that are fortified
* Fish, chicken, meat
* Eggs, peanuts, liver
* Wheat bran, seeds and nuts, seafood

* Fruits and veggies, lentils, beans, bran, peas
* Water with fluoride, some toothpaste and mouthwash
* Leafy greens, iodized salt
* Beef, Brazil nuts, quinoa, almonds, soybeans
* Tea, sweet potato, bananas, carrots, oats, tomatoes
* Kiwis, strawberries, peppers, broccoli, sunflower seeds
* Peanut butter, vegetable oils

Health Alert - Vitamin D is something your body needs to stay strong and healthy. By getting just 10 minutes a day of sun exposure without protection is approximately all a healthy adult needs. So yes, it's very important you lather up with sunscreen to protect your skin. But it's also good to give yourself a little bit of unprotected exposure to the sun each day. Your body needs this vitamin D to be healthy.

My Thinking . . .

Essential vitamins and minerals are going to help build your body and mind strong, and keep it that way. If you are suffering specific symptoms, it's important to speak with your doctor right away, because it could be a simple as adjusting a specific vitamin intake. For example, if you are extremely tired all the time you may have low iron stores. Increasing the amount of iron you are getting through diet really can make a difference. If this doesn't work, you may require a supplement. The end result will be an improvement in your overall health and well-being. That's worth its weight in gold.

50 Nutrition Pointers for Success in Health

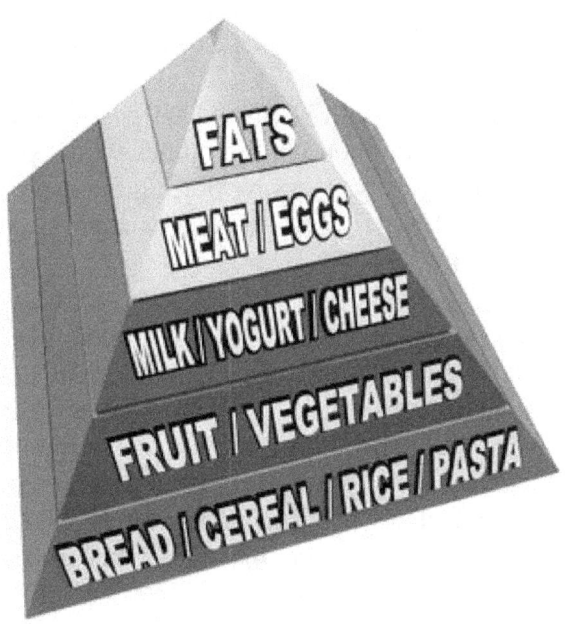

Bettering your health is something that you can always work on. It's not about going crazy and expecting to be "perfect" in your food choices out of the starting gates. That's not realistic for anyone, not even a trained athlete. The best route to successful health is the "one step at a time" approach. Arm yourself with the information you need to make better food choices and start applying.

Start small and work your way up, making sure you aren't too hard on yourself. You shouldn't feel guilty if you have a small piece of cake at a birthday party. But if you're still hungry, rather than go back for seconds, have a piece of fruit or maybe some whole grain crackers instead. This way you get to have your treat but not go overboard with it. This will take some time to learn but if you stick with it there will be positive chances in your health.

Here are a few pointers that will help you better your nutrition and most importantly improve your overall health.

* Fill your Cupboards with Healthy Choices - If you have sweet treats in your cupboards, then that's what you're going to eat. Set yourself up for success by putting healthier food choices within reach. This will make it easier for you to make healthy eating habit.

* Mini Meals Work Best - I know I mentioned this before, but eating smaller meals regularly throughout the day will help you lose weight and keep it off. It will happen faster too if your body can trust that you're going to feed it. It's time for you to mix things up and reprogram your body for the better. Offering it healthy fuel regularly is going to help level your mood, and curb your cravings. Two huge obstacles when it comes to eating.

* Easy on the Condiments - Try taking a step back and actually "tasting" your potato before you load on the fattening sour cream. Or maybe you want to take a bite of your fresh whole grain bread before slathering it with butter. Try these strategies for long enough and you will learn to enjoy them. They will become your new healthy normal, and the only thing your body is going to miss is all that fat you've lost.

* Cook without the Fat - You really don't need to fry your eggs in butter and oil for flavor. Spray a little Pam in the pan and season your eggs with salt, pepper, herbs and spices. This is going to save you hundreds of calories and oodles of fat that

would otherwise be clogging up your system. It's the little things that count.

* Bake, Broil, Barbecue or Steam - When you are cooking or ordering food in a restaurant. Opt for a lower fat cooking method just because you can. Deep frying is the one you really want to avoid because there is nothing good about it. The extra fat and calories you get when something is fried is absolutely crazy. Instead of having a piece of deep fried chicken you could have TWO pieces of grilled chicken for less fat and calories. More for less makes sense to me!

* Read Labels - I know this one can be pretty intimidating at first. But it's important to get into the habit of reading food labels. This way you know exactly what you are putting into your body, which makes it easier to make better food choices for you. Start by just looking at the calories and fat of the item you plan to eat. This is going to give you a strong base from which to build because if the calories are high along with the fat, you're best to steer clear of that food.

* Drink 6-8 Glasses of Water Daily - You've likely heard this one all your life and there's a reason. Water is essential to your good health. All of your body cells require water to function efficiently and effectively. Not getting enough water will leave you tired and without energy. Your skin and hair will lose their luster and your organs will be forced to work harder. Scientific studies have also shown people who deprive themselves of adequate amounts of water increase their risk of suffering a heart attack tremendously. Dehydration can be a very dangerous thing, so drink up!

* Keep the Table Clear of Serving Dishes - Research has shown that when food dishes aren't left sitting on the table people eat less food. This makes sense. So make sure you put the food on the plates and move the extras out of sight. It's only going to help.

* Easy on the Drinks - We tend to drink without thinking and this adds loads of fat and calories to your day. Did you know that a can of soda has over 300 calories and 8-10 teaspoons of sugar? Yikes! Juice drinks are also loaded with calories and fancy coffee drinks can contain more fat and calories than a whole meal. Sticking with pure water is best. Unsweetened herbal tea is great. And coffee and diet soda can be drank in moderation, just don't add loads of cream and sugar to your hot beverage. Drink smart here and you can cut out a whole lot of nutrition-less calories.

* Alcohol Beware - Alcohol is general chalk full of calories and sugars. The average serving of beer has 250 calories for instance. If you are popping back 2-3 an evening it really adds up fast. If you would like a beer, you should opt for a "lite" one. There are options that are as low as 67 calories a bottle. And steer clear of those fruity tropical drinks if you can.

A Long Island Iced Tea can have up to 780 calories! Margaritas are another to watch out for ringing in at 740 calories for just one drink.

If you are going to have a mixed drink, you're best to opt for a Run and Diet Coke, which comes in at just 65 calories. How about a Mike's Light Hard Lemonade with just 98 calories?

* Mix it up when Drinking Alcohol - Most of us have splurged on occasion with the alcoholic beverages. If you have water or diet pop between each of your alcoholic drinks, you're making a very good decision. Doing this is going to lower your total calorie count for the wild night out. It's also going to help re-hydrate your system so you don't have such a rough morning. Drinking alcohol dehydrates you and if you don't get the alcohol flushed out of your system, you're not going to feel so hot when it catches up with you.

* Take a Minute to Think About it - Studies have shown people who stop and consciously think about their last meal before they have a snack, they will eat few calories. This makes sense because many of us have conditioned to eat out of habit rather than need. Break this habit and you're going to drop fat and get healthy.

* Eat a small portion of protein at every meal – Researcher shows, that dieters who eat lean meat at every meal consume less calories overall. The theory is that protein fills you up longer, boosts metabolism, decreases cravings, and lowers your appetite.

* Pick Whole Grain Bread over White - Comparing the two, whole grain bread lowers your risk for various cancers and cardiovascular disease, and it leaves you fuller longer.
White bread really has no nutritional value and is going to give you a quick shot of sugar then send your energy levels straight down. Whole grains are going to level your blood sugars and help diminish those troublesome highs and lows we seem to experience daily.

* Experts Agree Fish is in - By eating fish twice a week you are going to sharpen your memory, improve vocabulary, and better your metal capacity. Speculation also is, that fish will naturally help lower the risk of developing Alzheimer's disease. It's definitely something to think about.

* Accountability - You may be a great independent worker. But having someone follow up with you regularly on your nutrition goals is only going to make your grass greener. Having someone constantly remind you of your nutrition goals and hold you to them is going to increase the chances of success. It's worth it, don't you think?

* Doggie Bag up Front - When eating out I can safely say the portion sizes are going to be WAY big. We are creatures of

habit and tend to eat what is on our plate, right? The solution here is to ask for a doggie bag up front and when your order arrives, put at least half into the doggie bag to have for lunch or dinner tomorrow. This way you can enjoy your restaurant experience without going overboard.

* All Electronics off - One reason many of us overeat is because we really aren't paying attention to what we're shoveling in our mouth. Turn off the television and your cell phone when you are eating, so you can tune into what your body is telling you. This will help you to keep from overeating and bring you one step closer to a healthier you.

* Chew Slowly - You've likely heard your mom or dad talk about this one. Taking the time to chew your food thoroughly is going to help you eat less. It takes time for your brain to connect with your stomach and communicate you're full. Slowing down your eating pace is going to teach you to realize when you're had enough, instead of overeating and figuring out after the fact you really didn't need that second hamburger.

* Plan Ahead - When you are looking to make better food choices, it's important to plan ahead. Please don't just "wing" it, because this is just setting yourself up to overeat. If you can plan your meals a week in advance that's the best option. But in the least, know what you are planning to eat one day before. This way you aren't going to just eat things here and there, while figuring out what to make for supper; not realizing till the end of the day you took in WAY too much.

* Keep a Food Diary - I know this one is a pain in the rear, but it's very important if you are serious about getting healthy with your food choices. A food diary is going to shock you into seeing how much you actually do eat each day. Usually this is loads more than your body needs. It's incentive to make changes if you will, and just knowing you are going to write down the handful of nuts you grabbed while making dinner, or

the ice-cream you finished up because your kid didn't, will help deter you from eating more than you need.

* If You're Really Hungry Eat Fruits/Vegetables - Studies have shown, people that normally eat more than five servings of veggies a day score higher on cognitive tests than those who don't. Another reason to eat healthy fruits/veggies is because they are generally low in calories and chalk full of fiber, essential vitamins and minerals. So they fill you up and give your body what it requires to function optimally.

* Green Tea Anyone? Researchers have found that green tea not only fights bad breath, but it also helps protect you from broken bones when you're older.

* Exercise before you eat - Studies have shown people that exercise just before eating consume less fat and calories. These people also tend to eat less throughout the day. Exercising does your body good.

* Get Your Sleep - Many people don't understand that adequate sleep each night is necessary for success in health. If you deprive your system of the shutdown time it craves, you're asking for trouble. Your body needs sleep to function optimally. Sleep directly affects how your body processes food, how much you eat, what kinds of food you eat and when, among other things. A sleep hormone called cortisol influences your sleep/wake cycle. It's often referred to as a "stress" hormone. People with high levels of cortisol tend to weigh more, eat fattier food choices, and overeat. Get 7-8 hours of sleep each night and your body will thank you for it.

* Don't Deprive Yourself - Your psychosomatic is important, and if you tell yourself you can't have a certain food, you're going to feel deprived. There isn't any one food you can't have. Just keep in mind moderation. So if you're at a birthday party and want some cake, have some. But why not share a piece

with someone, or just have a sliver instead of a slab. You can have a whole piece if you really want it, just add a half hour of cardio onto you gym routine the next day. Getting healthy in nutrition is a give and take relationship. When you figure out you have choice, you're going to be smiling big time.

* NEVER Skip Meals - I don't care what you've heard. Skipping meals is a "no-no" for everyone. What happens is your body actually shuts down on you because it doesn't trust you. When you do eat your body will try and store every bite of the carrot stick you give it as fat. I kid you not! Your metabolism will lower and you're going to burn even less calories no matter how much you exercise, or how little you eat. This may sound weird, but you've got to eat to lose weight. The idea is to eat healthier food choices regularly, but in smaller amounts. Add regular exercise to this and you're well on your way to better health.

* Stick to Simple - Food labels are confusing to say the least. Particularly if you pick up a package with a whole whack of ingredients, half of which you can't even pronounce. Just put the confusing package down and go for natural foods. A piece of fruit, low-fat yogurt, or whole grain crackers with peanut butter are the better choices. Simple is always the better choice when you're looking to make better food choices habit.

* Diversity is Key - We are creatures of habit. The same applies to our eating. We get used to specific foods and just seem to stick with them come hell or high water. By diversifying your menu, you're going to keep your body guessing for one. This is going to encourage your metabolism to kick it up a notch or two. Eating different foods will also deter you from getting bored with food. Boring eating can be VERY dangerous. You'll hit a point where control is lost in eating.

* Moderation Folks! - Moderation is key in anything you do. Too much of anything, including the good stuff, is NOT

healthy. Running is a fantastic cardiovascular activity to get your heart rate up, blood pumping, lose fat and flip your switch to positive. But if you are aren't training for a running event and are slipping on the sneakers and bolting 6 hours a day, that's too much! If you love playing video games and are now up to 12 hours a day every day, you are playing too much. The idea here is learning how to moderate yourself. With food, this is often a gynormous obstacle.

By teaching yourself to have 2 cookies instead of the whole bag, you're learning moderation. You don't need to slather half a pound of butter on your bread, or a whole bottle of full-fat salad dressing on your now unhealthy salad. Instead, just smear the butter and drizzle on about a tablespoon of dressing. There isn't anything you can't eat if you learn to adhere to moderation.

* Fruit and Juice Are NOT equal - Do not swap fruit juice for fresh fruit if possible. The majority of fruit juices are packed with sugar and additional additives to make it look pretty. Not to mention the fact the calorie count in fruit juices will shock you. Grab an apple, banana or orange, and if you are thirsty just stick to water. Your body will thank you for this.

* Take It All Off - The Skin That Is - Chicken skin in particular is loads of extra fat and calories you just don't need. Simply by removing the skin off your skin before eating, you can ditch at least a hundred calories of fat. It's one step in the right direction for sure.

* Break Dessert Habits - We program ourselves to eat what we eat. If you are expecting to eat dessert after each meal, you need to de-program this from your brain. This doesn't mean you can't ever have dessert again, because that would be silly. If you want dessert you can have it, but be smart about it. Maybe you want to make Friday's special and treat yourself to dessert. Or perhaps you want to always have dessert, but make

it healthier, or share it with someone. A bowl of fresh fruit topped with a touch of yogurt is yummy. Or how about baked apples with a sprinkle of cinnamon sugar? A lemon meringue cookie or even a couple of large marsh-mellows isn't going to throw you off course. Just understand that you really don't need a large piece of pie or chocolate cake after every dinner. This just isn't going to help you reach your health and wellness goals fast.

* Up Your Broccoli - Studies have shown that when eaten regularly, broccoli helps to protect against cancer. Broccoli is also a good source of calcium and numerous other nutrients your body requires to stay healthy and happy. Load up on broccoli and you are making a very smart move.

* Up Your Oranges - Oranges have been known to strengthen your immunity. People often up their vitamin C intake when they feel a cold coming on. Oranges are also fibrous and will help you eliminate harmful toxins from your system and support regularity. Grab yourself a little bit of juicy sunshine and see your body smile.

* Make Smart Snacking Easy - You are going to grab whatever's handy from the fridge when you're in a hurry. Set yourself up for success and make sure your cold zone is loaded with healthy choices. Yogurt, cheese strings, and fruits and veggies are a no brainer. Slice up for veggies for the week beforehand, so that when the munchies hit you can satiate them with healthy options. This doesn't mean you aren't ever going to crave unhealthy snacks. But at least this gives your head a chance to think about it before you gobble down the entire cake.

* Frozen Veggies are Fantastic! - Many foods frozen will lose their nutrients. When it comes to vegetables, this just isn't the case. In fact, frozen veggies are just as healthy as fresh ones, and talk about conveniently tasty! All you have to do is pop

them into the microwave and warm them up. Veggies are loaded with vitamins and minerals and make an awesome snack.

* Know your Numbers to Drop Pounds - There are 3500 calories in a pound. So if you want to lose weight and get healthy you are going to have to make sure you don't eat more than 3500 calories. In other words, you need to lower the number of fat and calories your body requires to maintain your weight, which you can do by making healthier and more nutritional food choices and incorporating exercise into your day. The best route for losing weight is to eat less and exercise more. The harder you work at this concept and the longer you stick with it, the more weight you will lose and the healthier you'll get.

* Choose Healthy Cuisine - There are some cuisines that are healthier than others in general. Indian, Thai, Chinese, Japanese, Mexican, and Greek are themes of food that are more likely to be healthy. Just keep that in mind when figuring out what foods to eat.

* Shop AFTER Eating - Many people don't even stop to think about this one. If you grocery shop when you're hungry, the chances of buying foods that are unhealthy increases tremendously. Instead, make sure you head to the market just after you've eaten, so that you aren't going to find yourself in a weak moment and head directly to the junk food isle. It does happen but try and make it the exception to the rule.

* One Bite Rule - This one may seem a little weird initially. First you must understand the way you eat has been learned. You have created your habits both good and bad. This means you have the ability to change them but it will take a whole lot of willpower, persistence and repetition. The "One Bite Rule," applies to those devilish delights we all love. Say you're out for dinner and usually have a decadent piece of triple chocolate cake with fudge drip icing. Allow yourself to have it, but put a condition on it. Take only one, maybe two bites, and leave it

alone. If you are eating with someone, maybe they'd be happy to eat the rest for you. If not, you can take your two bites and be done. You are teaching yourself the give and take relationship. Proving to yourself that you do have control over your actions and willpower to control what you eat. Are you going to screw up from time to time? Yes. Will it take a few more bites the first few times? More than likely. It's a learning curve and I don't expect you to be perfect, nobody is. But if you work at it you will more forward, and this "training of your thinking" is only going to help you get healthier and happier. Take it one step at a time.

* Steer Clear of Buffets - Buffets are just asking from trouble. At least initially they are. If you surround yourself with food and people that are eating everything in sight, it's really hard to not follow suit. Monkey see monkey do right? If you can help it, avoid going to buffets period. Just the same as making sure your cupboards aren't loaded with Ding-Dongs, chips and cookies.

Eventually when you are used to better eating choices, you'll be able to make out what you're going to eat and how much if you do happen to end up at a buffet. You haven't graduated to that stage yet though.

* Portion you Plate - It's naturally to feel more satisfied with more for the most part, wouldn't you agree? So fill your plate nice and full so that you feel like you aren't being ripped off. But make sure it's loaded with the right foods. Think of your plate like you would a clock. Load it with twenty-five minutes of fruits and vegetables, ten minutes of lean meat, fifteen minutes of complex carbohydrates, and ten minutes of low-fat milk products. This is just to give you the idea of what proportions of food groups you should be eating to help you set yourself up for success. If you've finished you meal and are still truly hungry, don't be afraid to have another serving of healthy vegetables. This will give you some extra nutrients and

fiber to help build your body strong without adding too many calories.

* Pre-Planning - It's really tough to keep your eating in check when you slip out to a restaurant, especially with friends. A trick that will help you keep control and make healthier food choices is to plan what you are going to eat before you head out. Have a look at the restaurant menu before you go, most are available online, and figure out what you are going to eat before you head out the door. This is going to help keep you on track, and if your mind is already made up before you get there, the chicken wings and battered shrimp aren't going to sway you, theoretically anyway.

* Mini-Meals Makes Sense - Your body doesn't have an on/off switch and is always burning energy. So it makes sense that you fuel it regularly and evenly. Most people are active during the day, and by spreading 5-6 smaller meals throughout the day at regular intervals, you're going to help your body burn more energy, keep energy levels up, avoid those dreaded afternoon lows, keep blood sugar levels stable, help you think clearer, and encourage fat to disappear. By eating regularly you are going to train your body to trust you and this is just going to help your body work more effectively and efficiently as a whole.

* Make a List and Check it twice - It's very important that when you are set to go grocery shopping, that you make a list. So you don't just buy what's on sale whether it is a smart food choice or not. Having a list whether it's written the old-fashioned way or typed into your Smartphone, will help you to buy what you need and not what you want. You will be focused on what you need to get, and this means filling your fridge and cupboards up with yummy-healthy instead of yummy-junky.

* Balanced Eating - It seems as if we are always looking for balance in our lives. When it comes to food, it's important to

make an effort to always eat balanced whether snacking, eating mini-meals, or having a regular meal. Strive to have the following in small amounts whenever you eat:

* Lean meat and meat products (protein)
* Healthy whole grains (complex carbohydrates)
* Low-fat milk and milk products (calcium)
* Fruits and veggies (essential vitamins and minerals)

An example might be a 6 whole grain crackers with a smear of peanut butter, a banana and a cheese string, or 3/4 cup of low-fat yogurt with half a cup of berries and half a whole grain bagel with a smear of jam. One portion grilled chicken (size of a deck of cards), 1/2 a sweet potato, a glass of milk and an apple will also work.

* Get Busy - Often when bored, we'll hit the snack cupboard. So theoretically if you keep yourself busy, you are going to set yourself up to back off on the treats. Instead of just sitting on the couch after supper why not go for a walk, join some sort of group, or find a hobby. Pick something that will keep you busy, and not with eating.

* Swap the Ice-Cream - Ice-cream is ok to have from time to time. But if you find yourself indulging a little too often, why not try swapping it for low-fat frozen yogurt? Give yourself time to adjust though. Don't expect to try "healthy" and crave it off the hop. If you stick with it, in time it will become your new habit treat - believe it!

* Chill - When it comes to making healthier nutrition choices it's not about being right or wrong, good or bad. What's important is that you give yourself a chance to make better choices. You aren't going to be perfect and need to accept this. Just recognize when you could have made a healthier decision and make it next time. Let your past decisions go, all eyes forward. Learn and just keep on learning and never give up. With

a little time and understanding you will make new healthier habits and you will see it's all worth it.

My Thinking . . .

Every single nutrition tip out there is going to help arm you with the information you need to make better health decisions for you. In this instance we are focusing on food. Some of these pointers you may find work well and are manageable for you. Others you might not be ready for yet, or perhaps they just don't apply in your circumstance. This doesn't matter because the information you gain from these tips can be stored and used to help you understand better nutrition and food choices in general.

Final Thinking . . .

Information is knowledge and knowledge is power. The wealth of nutritional information and methods of implementation are only going to empower you to reach your health and wellness goals with purpose. This book is all about making changes you can live with forever. It's about changes that take time, patience, understanding and perseverance. You shouldn't want it any other way if you are serious about improving your health and really WANT to learn how to make better nutritional choices that stick.

You now have the knowledge to take the first few steps in making it happen. Put one foot in front of the other and no looking back. You'll hit your goals just as long as you don't quit. Believe it!

Last Thoughts…

*THANK-YOU for reading my masterpiece. I hope you learned a little something, or at least got a few smiles.
*I would appreciate a millisecond or three of your time for a quick review, to help me build my masterful book empire higher.
*Whatever you do, don't forget to smile, and of course, check out my website for more of my e-Book masterpieces at: www.flawlesscreativewriting.com

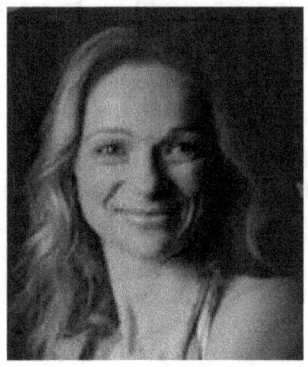

Cathy☺

www.ingramcontent.com/pod-product-compliance
Lightning Source LLC
Chambersburg PA
CBHW070458290526
45790CB00003B/1009